50 Things to Know

50 THINGS TO KNOW TO TAKE CARE OF A SPOUSE WITH DEMENTIA

Tales and Tips for Caring for Yourself and Your Loved One

Jessica Dumas

50 Things to Know To Take Care of a Spouse with Dementia Copyright © 2020 by CZYK Publishing LLC. All Rights Reserved.

All rights reserved. No part of this book may be reproduced in any form or by any electronic or mechanical means including information storage and retrieval systems, without permission in writing from the author. The only exception is by a reviewer, who may quote short excerpts in a review.

The statements in this book are of the authors and may not be the views of CZYK Publishing or 50 Things to Know.

Cover designed by: Ivana Stamenkovic
Cover Image: provided by the author

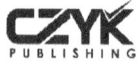

CZYK Publishing Since 2011.

50 Things to Know

Lock Haven, PA
All rights reserved.
ISBN: 9798578978449

50 THINGS TO KNOW BOOK SERIES REVIEWS FROM READERS

I recently downloaded a couple of books from this series to read over the weekend thinking I would read just one or two. However, I so loved the books that I read all the six books I had downloaded in one go and ended up downloading a few more today. Written by different authors, the books offer practical advice on how you can perform or achieve certain goals in life, which in this case is how to have a better life.

The information is simple to digest and learn from, and is incredibly useful. There are also resources listed at the end of the book that you can use to get more information.

50 Things To Know To Have A Better Life: Self-Improvement Made Easy!

Author Dannii Cohen

This book is very helpful and provides simple tips on how to improve your everyday life. I found it to be useful in improving my overall attitude.

50 Things to Know For Your Mindfulness & Meditation Journey
Author Nina Edmondso

Quick read with 50 short and easy tips for what to think about before starting to homeschool.

50 Things to Know About Getting Started with Homeschool by Author Amanda Walton

I really enjoyed the voice of the narrator, she speaks in a soothing tone. The book is a really great reminder of things we might have known we could do during stressful times, but forgot over the years.

Author Harmony Hawaii

There is so much waste in our society today. Everyone should be forced to read this book. I know I am passing it on to my family.

50 Things to Know to Downsize Your Life: How To Downsize, Organize, And Get Back to Basics

Author Lisa Rusczyk Ed. D.

Great book to get you motivated and understand why you may be losing motivation. Great for that person who wants to start getting healthy, or just for you when you need motivation while having an established workout routine.

50 Things To Know To Stick With A Workout: Motivational Tips To Start The New You Today

Author Sarah Hughes

50 THINGS TO KNOW TO TAKE CARE OF A SPOUSE WITH DEMENTIA

BOOK DESCRIPTION

Did you know that there are 5 million people in the US living with Alzheimer's and by 2050, there are projected to be 14 million? Spreading awareness of Alzheimer's and other types of dementia is desperately needed. There are many more people with these diseases than other diseases that get much more money approved for research from the government or from donations.

This book was written to bring better awareness that people with dementia matter. Plus, the self-sacrificing hardworking caregivers who take care of spouses also matter.

Having a spouse that you have loved for years begin to change because of dementia can be distressing. This book will help you by informing you of 50 or more things that will help reduce many of those scary and stressful feelings, as well as help you be more calm in situations you may be facing such as anger, delusions or misbeliefs, depression, unusual behavior, and more.

Some of the 50 or more things will be lessons learned from the author while she was caring for her husband and the rest will be from different resources. The author, Jessica Dumas, does not claim to be in the medical field but rather has an abundance of knowledge due to the experience of caring for her husband who had vascular dementia for almost five years.

Ask yourself if any of the following is a concern to you:
- Do you suspect that your spouse has some type of dementia?
- Has your spouse been diagnosed with a type of dementia?
- Are you apprehensive about what to do to be prepared for the future of caring for your spouse with dementia?

If you answered yes to any of these questions, then this book is for you...

50 Things to Know to Take Care of a Spouse with Dementia by author Jessica Dumas offers a more personal approach as well as being detailed and more understandable than many books. Much of the information in books or online is in clinical or medical terms. Although there's nothing wrong with that approach, it can be hard to understand. Instead of getting lost in the large amount of information on the internet, you can use this book as a research tool and a workbook. Jessica has written this book to help you not have to go through some of the awful experiences

that she did that could have been avoided if she would have had a book like this. The main objective of this book is to help you take care of your spouse as best you can. Jessica realizes what an exhausting, complicated, and tedious job you have and has given you 23 extra things or tips to help you with caring for your spouse.

In these pages, if your spouse has not found out that he/she has dementia, you will discover what the early symptoms are, why it is important to see a doctor early, doctor visit preparation, what tests will be done, and more. If you know your spouse has dementia and has been diagnosed with a certain type, this book will help with how to deal with denial, pulling together a Care Team with ways to get people to volunteer to help, hiring other caregivers, documents needed for a Care Plan to plan for the future, ways of handling situations like delusions, the different stages and their symptoms, links to several types of checklists and forms, plenty of resources, and much more.

By the time you finish this book, you will know at least 50 things to be able to give your spouse with dementia the care that is needed and that he/she rightly deserves…. So, grab YOUR copy today. You'll be glad you did!

TABLE OF CONTENTS

50 Things to Know
Book Series
Reviews from Readers
BOOK DESCRIPTION
TABLE OF CONTENTS
DEDICATION
ABOUT THE AUTHOR
INTRODUCTION
About Dementia
1. The meaning of dementia
2. Alzheimer's Disease (AD)
3. Vascular dementia
4. Dementia with Lewy bodies
5. Cause of dementia
6. Decreasing the risk of dementia
7. A helpful nutrient

Pay Attention to Small Changes
8. Paying attention to subtle changes
9. More time to do things together
10. Allows time for habit changes
11. Allows for starting medication that may help
12. Peace of mind knowing what's wrong
13. Time to enjoy abilities longer
14. Having more time to tell others

15. Having more time for research
16. More time for clinical trials
17. More time for legal arrangements

Seeing a Doctor with Early Symptoms

18. Other possibilities
19. Early symptoms to see a doctor about
20. Memory loss
21. Loss of words
22. Losing items
23. Social anxiety
24. Vision changes
25. Difficulty making decisions
26. Time confusion
27. Getting lost easily
28. Following directions
29. Lack of concentration
30. Judging distance
31. Mood, behavior, or personality changes
32. Denies impairment
33. Paranoia or fear
34. Sleeping problems
35. Lack of motivation

Seeing a Doctor

36. Preparing for a doctor visit
37. Notifying the doctor's office
38. Doctor checklist

50 Things to Know

39. How is dementia diagnosed?
40. Tests and processes for dementia

Finding Out What is Wrong

41. What the doctor says
42. Reaction to the news

The Care Team

43. Building a care team
44. Steps on getting a care team together
45. The Care Team meeting

The Care Plan

46. Making a care plan
47. Preventing preventative care
48. In-home professional care

Legal Decisions and Documents

49. Healthcare or advance directive
50. The DNR decision
51. Financial power of attorney (FPOA)
52. Know your spouse's wishes
53. End-of-Life Plan
54. Brain or body donation to science

Stages of Dementia

54. Early stage
55. Middle stage
56. Late stage

Caregiver Tips

57. Caregiver hotline

58. Caregiver mindset
59. Journaling
60. Caregiver Support Programs
61. Scheduling
62. Caregiver classes
63. Choosing medical and safety equipment
64. It is not personal
65. Something is not right
66. Taking breaks
67. Seeking other care
68. Taking care of yourself
69. Learning the language of love
70. Anger management
71. Handling misbeliefs or delusions
72. Be around family
73. The silver lining conclusion

Other Resources:

50 Things to Know

DEDICATION

This book is dedicated to:

- Robert H. Dumas Sr., my late husband of 30 years

- Gilmore Raphael, a dear friend of over 40 years

- All the persons who are living with dementia

- All the commendable persons taking care of those with dementia

ABOUT THE AUTHOR

Jessica Dumas was raised in the countryside near Stillwater, Minnesota. That is where her love of butterflies was born and has been carried throughout her life as a means of inspiration and motivation. Her love of butterflies inspired her to want to live in California where she could see butterflies all year long. Butterflies also inspired her to want to learn to fly. After marrying and having a daughter, she followed one of her dreams of moving to the Los Angeles area.

After being divorced from her first husband, she met Robert Dumas who was a flight instructor. He made it possible for her to fulfill the dream of learning to fly. Then somewhere between the takeoffs and landings, they fell in love and married. They had two boys together and along with her daughter, they would fly all over California, as well as taking several road trips across the country to see family and this beautiful country.

Jessica had a career in administration working as a document specialist for several industries including environmental and healthcare consultants. After leaving Corporate America in 2002, she was able to follow another dream of opening her own business called The Butterfly Connection. Her business as a Virtual Assistant kept her busy performing computer instruction and administrative support services.

Robert was 15 years older than Jessica and after he retired, he began suffering from strokes that caused vascular dementia. She took care of him for almost five years before his death in 2007. One year later she was diagnosed with early-stage breast cancer. She was told that the stress she endured caring for Robert contributed to the cause. After an operation and radiation, she has remained cancer-free. One reason for writing this book is her desire to help caregivers be aware that not taking care of themselves can cause health problems.

Some years later, Jessica was able to follow yet another dream of becoming a writer. Since 2017, she has written several eBooks that she has self-published. She has six books of her own on Amazon, as well as being able to write three books about butterflies as co-author, and several other nonfiction books as a ghostwriter.

Jessica continues to follow her dreams and is now in the process of fulfilling one of writing her life story. The eBook will be a novel series based on the life story of Robert and herself. She expects to publish the first edition of the series Butterfly Dreams with the subtitle of The 1st Generation—I'm Growing Wings, which will be on Amazon by March 2021.

Jessica now lives in a small mountain town north of Phoenix, Arizona. She continues to write for clients of her business and the freelancer website of UpWork.com. She continues her original passion for butterflies by being a monarch butterfly advocate, making butterfly jewelry, designing butterfly greeting cards and artwork, and writing poetry about butterflies, as well as other poems about nature.

You can read her three books of poetry, her book The Captain-A Memoir of Life with the Best Flight Instructor in LA County, as well as other pieces of work on her writer's portfolio website at www.jessicajdumas.com.

You can read her three books of poetry, her book *The Captain-A Memoir of Life with the Best Flight Instructor in LA County,* as well as other pieces of work on her writer's portfolio website at www.jessicajdumas.com.

Jessica has two Facebook pages. One is her personal page at https://www.facebook.com/TheButterflyConnection.

The other is called "Changes" where she displays butterfly-related poems and positive sayings on photos of butterflies to help people going through changes in their life at https://www.facebook.com/mybutterflyconnection/.

INTRODUCTION

> *"'You might be the scariest girl I've ever met,' he told her. 'Let's not be dramatic,' she said drily. 'I'm the only girl you can remember ever meeting.'"*
>
> — Sherry Thomas, The Perilous Sea

As we age, we have all made jokes about memory loss. Youngsters will tease parents and grandparents about it. Our friends may kid us about it. You may have a loved one that has had some memory issues and may have wondered if it is a sign of pending Alzheimer's. With all the stuff we put in our brains, it only makes sense that our brains can become overloaded especially if we are tired, stressed out, or not feeling well. However, if it goes on for some months without improving, you should be concerned and that's where this book comes in as it will let you know what to look for and what to ask the doctor about.

Unfortunately, we live in a society that sees the elderly and especially those with memory disorders/diseases as useless or crazy. The only way to stop this type of stigma or wrong idea is for you and everyone else to do what they can to make people aware that dementia is a disease they do not need to be afraid of.

When you volunteer to take care of your spouse, you become a dementia advocate as someone who wants to help find a cure. However, you may find that many friends and even family will fade away. This may happen due to them not knowing what to say to you or your spouse. It may be due to not wanting to be embarrassed if with your spouse in public. As far as I am concerned, any reason or excuse is not a good one.

Topics to be covered will be explaining exactly what dementia is and what types there are, early symptoms that should not be ignored, the initial doctor visit, how dementia is diagnosed or figured out after testing, getting together a care team and plan, legal documents, caregiver tips, and much more. I am writing this book to pass on what I have learned about dementia to help others who suspect their spouse may have it or that have a spouse diagnosed with some form of dementia.

There is a video on YouTube that can give you and others an excellent insight into what a person with dementia goes through. It is called "Experience 12 Minutes in Alzheimer's Dementia" and it made me cry. The link is in the Resources at the end of this document. Watching it before reading this book will help you see why your spouse will need help and why we must do much more to spread awareness.

There is a wealth of information in this book. You may already be overwhelmed by the responsibility of taking care of your spouse and I do not want you to get overwhelmed by all the information in this book, so take your time and read a little at a time. You will be glad to find that practically everything you need to know is at your fingertips.

ABOUT DEMENTIA

1. THE MEANING OF DEMENTIA

Dementia is the loneliest disease there is because people who have it do not have a connection with other people. Even though they have people around them, they lose the ability to connect in the way we normally do. Dementia is also known as a major neurocognitive disorder (both mental and nerve problems). The medical dictionary defines dementia as a condition that is usually progressive that has multiple cognitive or mental problems that did not originate from birth. The most common symptoms are loss of memory, loss of the ability to plan, loss of the ability to initiate actions or behaviors that are complex. Dementia is used as an umbrella term for all types of this condition such as Alzheimer's, vascular dementia, dementia with Lewy bodies, and ten others that are not as common.

The World Health Organization says that the number of people in the world with dementia is over 50 million. It is one of the hardest diseases for people to accept and the number one cause for losing independence. Before getting into the specifics of taking care of a spouse with dementia, it is important to know some facts about it such as causes, early symptoms, reasons to see a doctor early, etc.

The three most common dementia conditions are Alzheimer's, vascular dementia, and dementia with Lewy bodies. According to experts, ten other types of dementia consisting of Parkinson's disease, Wernicke-Korsakoff Syndrome, Creutzfeldt-Jakob Disease (Sometimes Called Mad Cow Disease), Frontotemporal Dementia (Pick's Disease), Huntington's Disease, HIV/AIDS Dementia, Fatal Familial Insomnia, Normal Pressure Hydrocephalus, Chronic Traumatic Encephalopathy/Brain Injury, and mixed dementia which can be a combination of different dementias. The three most common dementias are discussed next.

2. ALZHEIMER'S DISEASE (AD)

Alzheimer's is the 6th leading cause of death which starts out slow. In the early stage, short-term memory loss is common and other early signs as discussed later. As it progresses into the middle stage, it potentially gets worse with psychological and behavioral symptoms. In the middle stage, long-term as well as short-term memory is affected, making decisions are difficult, and irritabilities or anxiety become more noticeable. Sometimes sundowning (increased anxiety as evening approaches) is present and some may experience delusions, fear, and paranoia.

As it progresses into later stages, there may be inappropriate behaviors when in a social setting, withdrawal, having less desire to be with others, and the tendency to wander. There can also be a lack of personal hygiene, loss of appetite, loss of coordination and balance, sleeping difficulty, confusion, depression, and difficulty communicating (see Stages of Dementia for more detail). The order that the disease progresses is not the same with everyone so it can be hard to tell which stage is present with your loved one.

Scientists have found that AD is caused by high levels of molecules called plaques and tangles that cause lesions in the brain. Plaques are abnormal clusters of protein fragments that build up between nerve cells. Dead and dying nerve cells contain tangles, which are made up of twisted strands of another protein.

3. VASCULAR DEMENTIA

Vascular dementia is the second most common dementia and the easiest to diagnose since it is usually caused by having strokes. It can also be from changes in the brain such as white matter lesions and narrowing of the arteries. Early symptoms are like AD but will progress differently in a step-like way by progressing some and then stabilizing, but if another stroke strikes, it can get worse unless the strokes can be stopped. The person can live for several years and may improve somewhat. The cause of death is usually a stroke or heart attack.

4. DEMENTIA WITH LEWY BODIES

The third most common is called dementia with Lewy bodies which is like Parkinson's. It has body symptoms like Parkinson's such as motor and muscle weakness and rigidity or stiffness, as well as brain symptoms like difficulty making decisions, poor attention span, and memory loss. The body symptoms may start a year or so before the mental or at the same time but start slowly. There is confusion about the differences between dementia with Lewy bodies and

Parkinson's disease dementia. They are both types of Lewy body dementia.

Whatever type of dementia a person has, there is always the question of what caused it which is discussed in the next topic.

5. CAUSE OF DEMENTIA

Certain types of dementia have a definite cause such as vascular which is caused by a stroke that damages the brain. Dementia can start after mild strokes that do not cause the person to be disabled. Many other things can be factors such as old age, an accumulation of protein in the brain, repetitive injury to the head, infections with a high fever, heavy alcoholism or substance use, certain medications, low thyroid, genetic or family history, nutritional or vitamin deficiencies, tumor or cancer of the brain, pesticides or other poison, diabetes, heart or lung disease, and several other diseases.

While age certainly increases risk, it is not a direct cause of Alzheimer's. Age 65 is the most common onset age and with every five years, the risk doubles. The risk increases even more after age 85. AD is more of a risk if you have a close relative that has or had it. The most common risk factor is old age, but it is not the direct cause. Certain races of people have a higher risk such as Latinos and African Americans which is not understood but can be due to lifestyle or that vascular disease tends to be more common with them than the general population. Some things reduce the risk of getting dementia and is covered next.

6. DECREASING THE RISK OF DEMENTIA

Before we get into more things to know about dementia, giving you some suggestions on how to avoid dementia that should be noted for the benefit of yourself and other loved ones. Making such changes in your life as noted below may help decrease the risk or delay dementia if your spouse has it, and will benefit you and other family members so that you can avoid dementia in the future. Increasing age is the greatest known risk factor for AD and other dementias, but they are not a normal part of aging. The main things that will help decrease the risks of getting dementia include:

- Avoidance of excessive alcohol and tobacco
- Exercising both the mind and the body
- Having a healthy heart and other organs
- Being active socially with more than just social media
- Avoiding injuries to the head by protecting it with helmets during sports

- Avoiding injuries to the head by avoiding or leaving abusive relationships as quickly as possible.

- Eating healthy, including the food that increases ACh (see a helpful nutrient in the next topic)

7. A HELPFUL NUTRIENT

An interesting factor was discovered some years ago about getting the right nutrition to the brain. Acetylcholine (ACh) is a key neurotransmitter that scientists have identified as responsible for strengthening neural pathways and making new connections in the brain. Low levels of this neurotransmitter will cause dementia as the brain shrinks without being able to repair itself. However, some studies say a helpful nutrient is choline. We need it for the proper function of the nervous system, membranes around our cells including the brain cells, and to control muscles. The best way to increase ACh on a long-term basis is through regular exercise, taking supplements such as choline, or eating a diet that is rich in protein, eggs, omega-3 fish oil, beans, nuts, peas, and leafy greens. Unfortunately, there are several supplements advertised to increase ACh that could be scams. Before taking any supplement or giving any to your spouse, check with you and your spouse's doctors. Another thing to check with the doctor about is any signs that could be early dementia symptoms.

PAY ATTENTION TO SMALL CHANGES

8. PAYING ATTENTION TO SUBTLE CHANGES

When you have been married for several years, you get so used to seeing your spouse that you may not notice subtle changes. In the case of vascular problems, your spouse may have small strokes that are not obvious. My husband had been a heavy drinker and even though he quit, he was still having mild strokes that I did not notice until one day he said he could not get his fork to his mouth to eat. I then took him to the ER where they did a CT and saw that he had been having small strokes.

Even before that happened, there were subtle things that I dismissed. One side of his face was slightly drooping, but I assumed it was due to getting older since everything starts to droop. Us girls especially know about that! Another thing was that he had been getting upset with family members more than usual. He had always thought highly of his mother, but then started to talk bad about her and refused to talk to her. I thought that was strange but because he was an alcoholic, I figured it was his mood shifting as it had for years. However, it was a change in his usual behavior.

I want to point out that if your spouse displays any unusual mental symptoms that he/she did not have before, you need to get him to a specialist because his primary may not take it seriously. I am not sure if doing that would have saved my husband from having more severe strokes, but if you have noticed unusual behavior, it is worth checking into. The next nine topics will address reasons for getting an early diagnosis that will help you take care of your spouse.

9. MORE TIME TO DO THINGS TOGETHER

You and your spouse will be able to do some things that you may not be able to do later. Have you been thinking about going on a trip or having a special event such as a family reunion? Now is the time to do such things, so that you and your spouse can enjoy seeing the country or time with the family.

10. ALLOWS TIME FOR HABIT CHANGES

Your spouse will have some time to make changes in some habits that will prolong living such as quitting smoking, quitting alcohol, or getting into an exercise program. Your spouse can improve his/her memory and other mental functions by doing mentally challenging things to help stimulate the brain such as games or puzzles, reading, writing, as well as more socializing.

11. ALLOWS FOR STARTING MEDICATION THAT MAY HELP

Some medications and supplements help control or lessen some symptoms. Some medications help anxiety or depression. Other medications may help symptoms related to other diseases such as Parkinson's. The sooner they are administered to your spouse, the better he/she may feel mentally and physically.

12. PEACE OF MIND KNOWING WHAT'S WRONG

It may be helpful emotionally when your spouse is told why certain symptoms are happening. Most of us have a frustrating time when we do not know what is wrong with us. Even if the diagnosis is something you or your spouse do not want to hear, it will help you move on with your life.

13. TIME TO ENJOY ABILITIES LONGER

Your spouse would be able to make the most of his/her existing abilities. If your spouse was depressed and gets antidepressants, he/she may perk up and want to do more with hobbies or interests that they had lost interest in. He/she may even take up new hobbies or interests if encouraged to do so. My husband used to be an avid reader but as dementia got worse, he did not enjoy it, so I suggested reading to him and he loved that up until the day he died.

14. HAVING MORE TIME TO TELL OTHERS

Your spouse would be able to explain to family and friends what changes he/she is going through instead of you needing to explain it to them later. Some people with dementia are embarrassed to tell family and friends. That's understandable and you can encourage him/her by saying you can tell them together. You will have more time to get your Care Team and Care Plan created as well as asking people for help or hiring an in-home care provider as discussed later.

15. HAVING MORE TIME FOR RESEARCH

The sooner you know, the sooner you can do research and look for resources that may be of help later. There will be several unknowns to research and discuss with others which will take some time. It was helpful to me to keep a notebook on things I wanted to research and questions I had for the doctor or for searching the internet.

16. MORE TIME FOR CLINICAL TRIALS

There are always clinical trials going on for AD and other forms of dementia. The time your spouse must be eligible for taking part in a clinical trial will depend on the trial. Some clinical trials want people who have just been diagnosed and others may want different reasons to be eligible. Clinical trials can bring good outcomes.

17. MORE TIME FOR LEGAL ARRANGEMENTS

You and your spouse will have time to get a healthcare directive or living will complete. Other legal documents should also be done if not already such as a healthcare directive, End-of-Life Plan, or Last Will and Testament (see the Legal Decisions and Documents section).

Now that you have a list of early symptoms that should be checked out, the next section will go into when to see a doctor, tips for when you see the doctor, what tests may be done, and what to do after diagnosis.

SEEING A DOCTOR WITH EARLY SYMPTOMS

18. OTHER POSSIBILITIES

Some conditions can mimic dementia and it is important to see your primary doctor first when suspicious. Some people will have symptoms months or even years before a diagnosis of dementia is given. Some early symptoms may be dismissed by some doctors. Being proactive and keeping a journal on symptoms is important (see Journaling under Caregiver Tips). You will then have a documented history to show a doctor. You can also ask others if they see a difference in your spouse. One of the most common symptoms is social withdrawal. Since some people are naturally this way; however, you would be able to tell if this is an unusual symptom. Many times, persons do not see their symptoms so it will be up to you to take note that any early symptoms described below should be addressed with your spouse's doctor.

ND
19. EARLY SYMPTOMS TO SEE A DOCTOR ABOUT

There are early signs that should be checked out. Some experts say that if two or more are a concern, you should get your spouse to the doctor. But others say that if just one of the early signs is a concern, you need to get your spouse to the doctor. An important thing to start doing when you start noticing your spouse doing things or having behaviors that are not usual is to keep a record. We will cover keeping a journal and what to keep track of later (see Journaling under Caregiver Tips). There are differences of opinion from experts on how many early symptoms should raise a red flag, so I will list them all. The next 15 topics have been compiled on early signs from several expert websites.

20. MEMORY LOSS

Memory loss that causes disruption or concern by others is the most common early symptom of dementia. There can indeed be some memory loss as you age but it is usually not so significant. The type of memory loss to get checked out is the short-term type. Your spouse may repeat the same question or statement in conversation. Or your spouse may lose his/her train of thought and not be able to trigger the memory of what he/she was talking about. Your spouse may not remember something that happened a few minutes or hours ago.

21. LOSS OF WORDS

Forgetting words while talking or writing is an early sign that can be frustrating for your spouse. He/she may substitute a word or describe the word they are trying to think of in other terms. He/she may also use the wrong words without realizing it. It is common to not be able to think of names of places, things, or people especially while talking.

22. LOSING ITEMS

Misplacing things and not remembering how they got in unusual places is something your spouse may do. If he/she cannot find their cell phone, look for it in places like the refrigerator or a kitchen cabinet. Asking him/her to retrace steps will usually not help because their short-term memory loss will prevent them from remembering what they did a short time ago. This can be so frustrating for some who already have anxiety problems. If you can distract your spouse with some other activity that will help calm him/her down, you can then look for the item or wait until it turns up.

23. SOCIAL ANXIETY

Your spouse may become socially withdrawn when he/she was not before. It can be like agoraphobia which is the fear of leaving the house. You may need to coax your spouse to get him/her to go anywhere. This usually happens because the person gets embarrassed about how he/she is feeling when around people. Sometimes another person will be able to persuade him/her to go to a social occasion better than you can.

24. VISION CHANGES

If your spouse complains about unusual vision problems that are not the usual ones as before, this could be a symptom. Some changes may be things such as not seeing colors or contrasts. An eye doctor would be able to tell if this may be an early symptom.

25. DIFFICULTY MAKING DECISIONS

Not making decisions well as to how to dress for certain weather conditions is common. Your spouse may put on shorts in the winter or a warm shirt in the summer. He/she may be having a decline in personal grooming habits such as showering or shaving. It usually is because they do not remember when to do it or could be feeling uncomfortable such as being too cold to shower or some other reason.

26. TIME CONFUSION

Being confused about what day it is can be normal as one ages especially after retiring from working where you need to know what day it is. However, it is usually temporary and can be recalled within a few minutes. If your spouse cannot recall what day it is or what the month, year, or season is, this is an early symptom.

27. GETTING LOST EASILY

Depending on your spouse's experience with navigating in the past will determine if this is an early symptom. Getting lost easily when your spouse did not have this problem before is a red flag. This can be concerning if your spouse still drives by himself. You may have had to look for him/her while going shopping or doing other errands where you live. He/she may get disoriented while driving or walking. If the surroundings are ones your spouse has known for a long time, this can be an early symptom. This symptom can manifest itself as getting lost when wandering away in later stages.

28. FOLLOWING DIRECTIONS

Difficulty with things that take more than two or three steps can be an early sign. Examples would be following recipes, instructions for assembling something or playing certain games like cards. If it is anything that your spouse had no trouble with before, it should cause concern and be checked out.

29. LACK OF CONCENTRATION

Unable to concentrate for long or solve a problem can be an early sign. Examples would be difficulties making a shopping list, organizing items, planning an outing, comprehending what is read. These could also be signs of attention deficit disorder so it should be checked out.

30. JUDGING DISTANCE

This can be an early symptom if your spouse had no trouble with it before. He/she may trip easily when going up or down steps. What can also be disturbing is when your spouse may do such things when driving as hitting or rubbing curbs often and driving too close to others. It would be best for you to do the driving to avoid accidents.

31. MOOD, BEHAVIOR, OR PERSONALITY CHANGES

If your spouse previously had a quiet and mild-mannered personality, but then becomes loud or gets angry much easier than before, it could be an early symptom. Any drastic behavior change can be a sign. Some other early signs may be depression as well as being elated for no reason. Also, you should be aware that if your spouse is depressed, he/she may even become suicidal.

32. DENIES IMPAIRMENT

Anosognosia is a term used for when someone with dementia does not recognize their impairment which can happen at early and later stages. Your spouse may try to convince you that he/she is feeling fine. He/she may even accuse you of making up things about them.

33. PARANOIA OR FEAR

Your spouse may start thinking such things as someone is trying to hurt them or that the authorities are after them. He/she may accuse you of taking things from them if they cannot find them. He/she may become overly fearful of certain things that they were not afraid of before.

34. SLEEPING PROBLEMS

Some problems sleeping may be normal as you age, but they are typically temporary. If he/she has problems for several months such as not being able to go to sleep or stay asleep, it may be an early sign. Your spouse may start staying up all night by perhaps watching TV and then sleeping during the day. Getting days and nights mixed up can be an early sign.

35. LACK OF MOTIVATION

Depending on how motivated your spouse was before, if he/she shows signs of not being motivated to do things they enjoyed before, it could be an early symptom. He/she may display a lack of motivation when not being able to easily start a new project or losing interest in hobbies they used to like.

Any of the symptoms above should be checked out and especially if your spouse has more than one or two symptoms. Early symptoms can carry into later stages that are discussed in the Stages of Dementia section. Next, we will discuss tips for when seeing a doctor.

SEEING A DOCTOR

36. PREPARING FOR A DOCTOR VISIT

Now that we have covered symptoms that should be checked out, it is time to get your spouse to the doctor. This may be easier said than done. If your spouse is one of those that do not want to go to the doctor, make the appointment for them. When the time comes, simply say it is time for your check-up appointment as it is not necessary to say what exactly it is for. It is not necessary to try to get your spouse to understand why it is important to get an early diagnosis if they have any kind of dementia. If you must make up something to get them to the initial appointment, go ahead.

37. NOTIFYING THE DOCTOR'S OFFICE

If your spouse is having difficulty wanting to see the doctor, make it a point of telling the doctor's office staff, or nurse before the appointment that your spouse is not cooperative, and they will know how to handle it. You can also ask for the email address to send a breakdown of your spouse's behavior, and what you want your doctor to know privately. That way the staff will be ready. It is a good idea to call the morning of the appointment to confirm everyone is aware. If the doctor refers your spouse to a specialist, be prepared for more resistance and ask the doctor for suggestions on how to handle it. Remember that the diagnosis and doctor visits are more for you since you will be the one in charge of your spouse's care. Next is a checklist to take with you to the doctor's visit.

38. DOCTOR CHECKLIST

Below is a list of what to prepare for on your spouse's doctor appointment:

- Make a symptom list and include anything that you may not feel is related to dementia
- Include how often the symptoms happen and how long they last
- Make a list of all medications that your spouse is taking including any over the counter items such as vitamins and supplements along with the dosage
- List any life changes or stressful events that have happened recently
- List all your questions

Going with a positive attitude will help your spouse face the challenge. The doctor will consider all and then proceed with their ways of determining if there is reason to believe your husband should see a dementia specialist as discussed next.

39. HOW IS DEMENTIA DIAGNOSED?

First, the primary doctor can check if symptoms may be from something other than dementia by running blood work for such conditions as low thyroid, lack of certain vitamins, and other things that can affect the brain. If the doctor thinks more tests should be run, then they can refer your spouse to a specialist. A Neurologist specializes in the brain and nervous system and some tests can be done by a mental health specialist such as a psychiatrist or neuropsychologist (handles both neurological and psychiatry). AD now has biomarkers to make a diagnosis more accurate. The following are tests and procedures to determine dementia.

40. TESTS AND PROCESSES FOR DEMENTIA

Unfortunately, there is not one certain test that tells if a person has dementia. It is more like a process that the doctor will do to gather information about symptoms. It is important that you go with your spouse and be with him/her during testing, if possible.

If there are other caregivers or close family, ask them to also come to the appointment. After doing a medical and family history, a cognitive analysis is done to see how your spouse's memory is operating, what their abilities are in doing such things as communicating, counting, and reasoning. There are standard cognitive tests that include such things as drawing a picture of a clock with the hands of a clock showing a certain time, drawing certain shapes, doing simple math, counting backward by sevens, and other questions.

The doctor will question you and your spouse about symptoms which include not wanting to be around people, anger or being mean, depression or sadness, anxiety or nervousness, misbeliefs or seeing/hearing things not there, acting lazy or bored, being overly happy, irritated easily, shyness or the opposite, and unusual body movements. There are also neurological tests that will check your spouse's reflexes, balance, eye movements, and other senses such as smell since certain types of dementia can cause a loss of being able to smell.

Your doctor may refer your spouse to a psychiatrist or a neuropsychiatrist which is a specialist that evaluates how diseases of the nervous system contribute to mental disorders. Either one can do evaluations of moods, depression, anxiety, unusual behaviors, and the relationship your spouse has with you and other in the family. The doctor may ask about how often your spouse does things of concern and how long they last. This is where having a journal will come in handy.

Brain scans should be done using a CT or MRI to see if your spouse has had any strokes and to rule out any tumors. A PET (positron emission tomography) scan is a special X-ray machine that is useful in determining brain activity and if a certain protein called amyloid is present which will indicate if your spouse has Alzheimer's.

It may take weeks of testing and consultations to determine if your spouse has dementia. The next topic will discuss getting a diagnosis or doctor's report on what he thinks is wrong.

50 Things to Know

FINDING OUT WHAT IS WRONG

41. WHAT THE DOCTOR SAYS

If the doctors do not find enough evidence of dementia, it does not mean that he/she may not be diagnosed in the future so follow-up if any new symptoms appear. The doctor may refer you to a medical social worker or dementia advocate for assistance in the next steps. They are experienced and skilled at coordinating all the different aspects of coping with dementia. Many wonderful resources are available for people with dementia, and social workers know where the resources are and how to access them. They can help reduce the stress and anxiety of trying to make sense of all the changes and challenges brought on by dementia so that you can focus on living a quality life. The next topic goes into reactions to the diagnosis.

42. REACTION TO THE NEWS

Dementia will cause many changes in your life and coping with the idea can be a big shock for both you and your spouse. It is a good idea to take some time to let it sink in. Being aware is not the same as letting anxiety take over so that you jump right on taking care of things that need to be addressed and get everyone else in a panic. If you are feeling overwhelmed, that is when having family and friends to talk to is helpful.

Your spouse may have different reactions to the news. Many go into denial as it is just too much to imagine. Other reactions can be anger, guilt, resentment, and depression. Perhaps your spouse finds it easier to deny the disease than to deal with the awful truth. Since dementia can lessen being able to understand things, it can cause them to have a harder time accepting it. Problems with managing daily life can become a fight with your spouse when they cannot accept help or practice safety precautions. Try to get him/her to take it easy for a while by not going out to limit the chances of falling or other accidents until you can get some help.

Talking to your spouse about it may not be good for them unless they bring it up and want to talk about it. I remember how I used to try to explain what is happening to my husband's brain and I would get a blank stare like he was not comprehending it and then he would seem more depressed, so I quit doing that.

Your spouse may not understand what the diagnosis means so take some time with him/her and do some activities you enjoy. You may find that because your spouse wants to know about his/her condition that you go into too much explanation that can be confusing for them. How much you tell him/her should not depend on how much they want to know.

It will depend on how much you feel he/she needs to know.

Dementia is like the elephant in the room! But you can help make friends with that elephant by distracting your spouse so as he/she will not think this diagnosis is a death sentence and that life is over. Even though it is true that his/her life may be shortened, you do not know for sure by how much or what exactly the future holds. If you make it seem less of a problem and do not argue with his/her denial, he/she may be calmed by your suggestion and stop worrying. Depending on how believable you are and how much he/she understands about his/her condition, the following may be a way of helping your spouse accept it.

- Tell him/her you want to have a chat at a time he/she is most alert

- Calmly ask him/her to listen to what you are worried about

- Tell him/her that you are concerned because he/she is not getting enough vitamins (this would not be a lie since certain vitamins can help)

- Tell him/her how not getting certain vitamins can cause such things as some of the symptoms he/she may be experiencing like memory loss or trouble sleeping

- Ask if he/she wants the problem to get better which he/she most likely will

- Then tell him/her how worried you are about it and that you hope he/she will go to the doctor so he/she can get some vitamins.

This approach should have a calming effect. Some people with spouses diagnosed feel they do not want to tell anyone until it becomes obvious. That was my initial reaction, but then I realized that I was hurting him by keeping it a secret. Once people knew, I could then determine who may be of help. Having someone who is experienced with dementia is important since your spouse may listen to someone else better than you.

If your spouse is looking for something that will make him feel useful, there is the Alzheimer's Association National Early-Stage Advisory Group, which consists of people in the early stage of the disease who are helping raise awareness about dementia. Your spouse may be interested in joining this to give him/her some purpose (see link in Resources for the link). Another thing that will help your spouse is getting a Care Team together and then making a Care Plan as covered next.

THE CARE TEAM

43. BUILDING A CARE TEAM

According to Alzheimer's Association, having a Care Team can keep your stress level down for when issues come up that you do not know how to handle or there is an emergency, as well as the day-to-day issues. Having a Care Plan to go with the Care Team will be worth the effort and it should be on the top of your list of things to do after a diagnosis of dementia. People to ask to be on the Care Team would be people you trust, and your spouse would feel comfortable with. Others can be helpful in other ways.

If you need some time to figure out what you want everyone to do, simply ask if they are willing and available to help. If they agree to help, then you can tell them you will be planning a get together for everyone to let them know about what the doctors are saying, what tasks you will need help with, and that you will be sending them an invitation soon (more on that later).

The following may look like an overwhelming amount of stuff to do, but I tried to include as many details that are my suggestions, as well as those from resources online. Some will be things you may already know.

A Care Team can include the following persons:

Family/friends:

- Immediate family members that live with you or live close by
- Family members living farther away to be helpful on the phone
- Close friends of yours or your spouse

Professional members:

- Your primary doctor, general practitioner, and/or nurse practitioner
- Medical social worker, your insurance caseworker, or dementia advocate
- Specialists such as a neurologist, neuropsychiatrist, and/or others especially when other conditions exist

In the community:

- Neighbors you know
- Community organization members such as the local Community Center
- Social group members such as clubs you or your spouse belong to
- Members of your church or other local spiritual organization

44. STEPS ON GETTING A CARE TEAM TOGETHER

Getting a care team together may seem overwhelming, but if you have experience in planning a party or other group event, this will be like that, along with time spent in preparation, follow-up, etc. It would be good if you could get a social worker, advocate, therapist, or task manager set up before proceeding. This way they can be included in the meeting if they are able. Alzheimer's Association's website has support groups listed in your area that can help find appropriate professionals if your doctor has not referred you to any.

This is where your best friend or close family member comes in to be of help. They are the first ones to tell about your spouse's diagnosis and how much you will be depending on them to help. If you only know of a few people who may help, look at the below for ideas.

Make a list of prospective Care Team members by considering the following:

- Recruit a friend or family member to help you with the list
- Think of individuals who care and are willing to listen

- Avoid people who seem judgmental, critical, or blaming
- Make the list divided into two parts, one for those you know well enough to feel they will be of help, and one for those that are questionable
- Leave room after each name to make notes
- If you expect the list to be longer than ten people, use a computer to make a table in Word or use Excel (or have someone else do it)
- List everyone's phone and email
- If you are not sure of contact information for your spouse's friends/family, use his/her cell phone to get contact information
- List each doctor, specialist, social worker, and other professional
- List all others such as neighbors, groups or clubs, church members
- For those you do not have contact info on, you could visit neighbors to get info, go to a meeting with groups and collect contact information from some

members who can help or post a bulletin with them

- Take a preliminary count of how many may come

45. THE CARE TEAM MEETING

If the count of who may come to a meeting is small, you may choose not to do the following; however, I wanted to include it for those who have several to contact because even though it may seem like more work, in the long run, it will be easier. You may want to recruit a good friend or family member to help with these steps such as calling or emailing people, maintaining a list, sending thank you cards, or anything else. Having everyone get together has some benefits such as:

- They will get to see your spouse and how he/she is doing
- You will not need to repeat yourself several times
- You can have the meeting online with Zoom or Skype (everyone will need internet and email access)
- Or you can have it in person at a place with enough room such as at the local Community Center, apartment building

or neighborhood recreation room, or a restaurant so people can have lunch

If you decide on doing it in person, here are suggestions of details:

- Schedule the meeting
    - Once you decide on a place, choose a date and time within the next few weeks that you think would work for most people (weekday or weekend?)
    - Make an estimated count of how many may come
    - Call to reserve the meeting place – if at the Community Center
- Ask what kind of equipment they have for showing a video
- ii. Ask for the menu on that day and check if you can request certain items for a large group
- iii. If they can, have in mind what you want to be served and ask what they charge for individual lunches (a low price).
    - If at a restaurant meeting room, ask the same.
    - If unable to get a place that has a low-cost lunch and enough room, you can

50 Things to Know

always have it in your back yard or at someone else's house.

- Contact everyone on the list

  o Ask a family member or friend to help you do the calls/emails or mail invitations

  o Create, have someone else create, or purchase invitations for mailing.

  o Send invitations to those you have addresses for or email them – tell them about the meeting with directions to get there, why you are having it as well as what lunch will cost them; ask RVSP a week before

  o If you have no email or address but have a number, call and you can ask them then about helping or ask for an address to send an invitation.

  o When you get RSVPs, note on your list how many plan to come

- If they do not respond within a few days, send/call a reminder

- ii. If the count is considerably more or less than the original estimate, you may need to change your reservation

- For those who cannot come:
  - Ask if they are willing and available to help; if so, send the form
  - ii. Give them a general idea of what they can do to help, and let them know you will be contacting them later to give specifics
    - For doctors or other professionals, you can call their office or send an email saying you wish for someone to be on your spouse's Care Team and ask if anyone could come to the meeting to explain dementia.
- Before the care team meeting
  - Create a "Volunteer Sign Up" to list tasks you will need volunteers for indicating when/how often they can help (or have someone create and make copies) to give everyone at the meeting.
- Note on the form to watch "Experience 12 Minutes in Alzheimer's Dementia" before the meeting (Resources has link). It should encourage them to come and to help.
  - Fill out "This Is Me" form to that has your spouse's photo, background, likes, dislikes, achievements, routines,

any physical problems, etc. (see Resources for a link):

- Make copies to give to those who are definite volunteers or anyone who may be around him/her often such as a driver, therapist, social worker.

    o If a professional said they would come, call to confirm and ask if they will need any video equipment or anything else.

    o If not having at home, see if the place has video equipment or a smart TV so that you can show a presentation or video from a laptop. If you are not familiar with how to do this, ask friends/family to handle it.

    o Prepare what you want to say and if you're not able to show the above video, prepare to talk about it and remind them to watch.

- At the meeting
    - If a professional person is present, have them explain the diagnosis and other important facts about your spouse's condition.
    - Ask everyone to think about what they can do to help while having some refreshments or lunch.
    - Hand out the questionnaire form for them to volunteer for helping.
    - Collect all the forms and tell everyone you will be in contact with them; for any people that volunteer, give them the "This Is Me" copy; make a note on their volunteer form that they got the copy so you do not have to send later.
    - Ask if anyone has questions; make a note of questions you may need to research and let them know you will get back to them.
    - Have some fun socializing with your spouse being the center of attention.

- After the meeting
  - Call those who did not say they could volunteer to help at the meeting:
- Make it clear the type of help you may need now or in the future.
- ii. It may help with some if you suggest doing things together such as shopping or cooking.
  - If someone wants to help but is unable at the time:
- Ask them to let you know if that changes.
- ii. Ask if they know of someone that may be available. They may suggest someone you forgot to ask.
  - Express your appreciation
- Sending a thank you card with what they said they would do to help is a good way to remind them as well as thank them. Send a copy of "This Is Me" if they do not have it yet.

This may take some time to get completed, but it is important to get together as soon as possible. Now that you have a Care Team, the next topic will cover making up a Care Plan which you can also get help with preparing.

THE CARE PLAN

46. MAKING A CARE PLAN

Something you should know before I proceed is that making up a Care Plan may involve a good number of documents and keeping them organized can be a headache. To help you from pulling your hair out, I found a great document that helps you organize all the other documents. It is called Caregiver Document Organizer and you can download it from the National Caregiver Library that has a link in the Resources.

Deciding how you will proceed before things get worse is important. Believe me, it is better to be prepared at least to some degree. Dementia experts advise that people with dementia should have a Care Plan that is ongoing and gets updated at least once a year. This should not be confused with the Daily Care Plan discussed later which is somewhat like a schedule of things that your spouse does daily. A Care Plan is for all persons on the Care Team to assist them in knowing who all is on the team, what they are expected to do in certain situations, medications, and anything relevant to the care of your spouse.

Your spouse's doctor should be familiar with Medicare's coverage of care planning. If you have other insurance than Medicare, you can check with them as to coverage. Or you can get information about it at the Alzheimer's Association website (alz.org/careplanning). Care planning should include the following:

- The main caregiver, other caregivers, and all Care Team members

- The agent or person who is responsible for carrying out your spouse's medical decisions and who is the secondary person for what is called a healthcare directive or living will (see Getting a healthcare directive)

- Record your spouse's mental and physical abilities (see "This Is Me" below)

- Listing and recording how many and how long symptoms last (see Journaling).

- Listing medication taken and those to ask the doctor about

- Checking for safety factors to lessen chances of falls and accidents, including if your spouse should quit driving

- Checking to see and listing what medical equipment may be helpful

- Listing ways to help your spouse with organizing his/her world

- Listing caregiver needs and schedule (see Scheduling in Caregiver Tips).
- Choosing community services such as at a Community Center and other resources for both your spouse and you as a caregiver
- Choices for finding an in-home caregiver that does it for a living (see In-home professional care)
- End-of-life planning, including your spouse's wishes or things that help your spouse's quality of life and decisions on the type of hospice care to have.
- Filling out a "This Is Me" form or one like it to give to persons that will have contact with your spouse that has information about your spouse's personality and things they like, etc. (See Resources for a link to this document)

You can do a Care Plan without going online if you prefer but this service is a great help. Part of the quality of life in the Care Plan should include what type of care could be stopped.

47. PREVENTING PREVENTATIVE CARE

If your spouse is in the middle or later stages, do you insist on him/her going to all preventive exams? Some would be such as repeated lab tests or mammograms which may not be wise to continue. If your spouse gets highly upset at being stuck with a needle or being manipulated for certain exams, think about what would happen if they came down with some type of cancer. They would need to have a needle biopsy and then perhaps chemo and radiation. It would be difficult to put them through all that. You need to consider what you would do if your spouse needed several treatments that they would fight through and maybe even hurt themselves trying to get away from. It all depends on how far dementia has progressed. Try not to think about how you want them to live as long as possible, but rather what quality of life they will have during the time they have left.

There are choices you can make when it comes to who will care for your spouse. The next topic covers options.

48. IN-HOME PROFESSIONAL CARE

You may not be able to do all the work needed or get enough help from family or friends. You can hire an in-home care person through a home health agency or as an individual care provider. If you are not sure which is best, you should first see if both are covered under your insurance. Then seek opinions from other caregivers in support groups or community services. Medicare and other insurances will cover certain in-home health care services but only when your spouse is eligible. Usually being homebound and needing the reasonable services of a skilled professional will qualify him/her. You can call Medicare or other insurance you may have to find out for sure what they cover.

It can be difficult to find a care provider that you are happy with or that your spouse is happy with so below are some things to consider from Alzheimer's Association:

- Make a list of what care is needed for your spouse (filling out the form mentioned at the end of this topic can help)

- Call and ask what kind of help they provide to see if they will meet your needs and if so, set up an appointment for an interview in your home

50 Things to Know

- Prepare questions for your interview with them
- Ask a friend or family member to be with you to discuss your impressions afterward
- Meet with the prospective home care agency or provider and have them meet your spouse if you feel they may work out
- Get them to fill out an application with references
- Some questions you can ask are:
- Do you know how to do CPR and first aid?
- What experience do you have with dementia?
- How do you manage specific health and behavioral care?
- Do you have any special training in dementia care?
- Are you bonded? (important for potential losses)
- What kind of references do you have?
- What is your availability for the times we need?
- Who fills in for you if you are sick?

- Discuss with your friend or family member what they think of the person

- If going through an agency, check if they do a criminal background or if you need to do one; if an independent caregiver provider, you may need to do as well as prepare an independent contractor agreement so nothing is misunderstood (see Resources for a link to a website that you can pick your state and then fill in some information and download free).

- Call references for work history, experience level, any complaints, etc.

- Once you make a selection, get them familiar with your spouse's likes, dislikes, hobbies, activities, personal facts, and anything relevant.

You can download an 8-page form on Alzheimer's Association called "Our Personal Facts and Insights" as well as the "This Is Me" form (see link in Resources) to fill out on your spouse to help you organize and share information about personal preferences and background. This form is also good to give to any alternate volunteer caregivers and family. Part of the Care Plan is making legal decisions and getting legal documents made up as discussed next.

LEGAL DECISIONS AND DOCUMENTS

49. HEALTHCARE OR ADVANCE DIRECTIVE

A healthcare directive is also known as a living will, an advance directive, or a healthcare power of attorney. The purpose of a healthcare directive is to let your spouse document that he/she selects you as his/her healthcare agent to make medical decisions for them. If you do not already have such a document for your spouse, now is the time to get it. If your spouse is competent, he/she can express wishes for any important healthcare decisions that may arise.

One important thing is that your spouse can indicate his/her choice in being resuscitated if his/her heart stops or if not able to breathe on his/her own. This is called "do not resuscitate" or a DNR order as discussed next. The healthcare directive can also have other information that your spouse wishes such as not wanting any blood transfusions for religious reasons or not wanting any other medical procedure.

50. THE DNR DECISION

Many people believe that they would not want to be brought back to a life that has no quality and wishes to die naturally without being on any life support. A DNR can be part of the healthcare directive and may have a question to answer as to wanting a DNR or not. This will act as a legal order to stop any attempts at reviving your spouse, such as if CPR or defibrillation is used to prolong his/her life. If your spouse does not want to undergo CPR or advanced cardiac life support, it will be necessary to have a DNR choice completed on the healthcare directive that should be given to all your spouse's doctors. If you need the form, the doctor may have it, or you can download it from the internet at a website such as at eForms.com which will ask you to select the state you live in as different states have different laws regarding DNRs.

Without a DNR order, medical professionals would be required to do resuscitation procedures to keep your spouse alive. A DNR would not affect any treatment other than that which would require intubation or CPR. Patients who are DNR can continue to get chemotherapy, dialysis, or any other appropriate treatments. There are other legal documents to consider as covered in the next topic.

51. FINANCIAL POWER OF ATTORNEY (FPOA)

You may wish to have an FPOA also drawn up to give you the right to take care of all financial affairs for your spouse. Even though in most states each spouse automatically has this right to take care of financial matters concerning them both, it is a good idea to have one in place in case there is any property or accounts that are in your spouse's name only. You can find out more about this from a financial advisor or attorney. You can also download this type of FPOA from the internet, but make sure it is for your state. The next topic covers knowing what your spouse's wishes are about the end of his life.

52. KNOW YOUR SPOUSE'S WISHES

In my case, my husband got pneumonia near the end of his life and the doctors said he would continue to get pneumonia from aspirating his food because he had a stroke that affected his throat and breathing. He would choke sometimes, and I had to start feeding him because he would take big bites and then choke. The doctor told me that the best thing was to insert a stomach tube to feed him. I asked him if he wanted a tube in his stomach and he emphatically said, "No!."

I knew this would shorten his life, but I had to consider what I would have wanted if it were me and the answer was the same. He was then transferred to hospice and ate the soft food they provided. He improved for about a week, so several of his 11 children and their families were able to visit him for the last time and he enjoyed his last few weeks. I never regretted that decision but if I would have had a Care Plan in place, it would have gone much smoother and timelier as I would have had his approval beforehand.

My point in telling you my story is that knowing what your spouse would prefer ahead of time can save time and anguish. The way to know what he/she prefers is to do an End-of-Life plan which is part of the Care Plan and discussed next.

53. END-OF-LIFE PLAN

An End-of-Life Plan consists of the wishes, arrangements, and treatment selections that your spouse would want at the time shortly before death and after. When there is not an End-of-Life Plan in place, you and other families need to make all these decisions after he dies. Sometimes these wishes are put into a Living Will, but I find that the End-of-Life Plan is much more detailed.

You can make these decisions without his/her input but if your spouse has any preferences such as to be cremated instead of buried or has other wishes, he/she should have a part in making up this document. Even though I did not have a plan in place, I still knew most of his wishes. The way I handled this was to ask him questions one at a time in a casual way. There is no need to drag him down to the attorney's office to make out all the End-of-Life Plan documents unless he/she is normally the financial/business person in the family and still is competent enough to do this. An End-of-Life Plan includes such things as below:

Selection of you as Appointee and an alternate who would be responsible for carrying out or executing your spouse's wishes

Where he/she prefers to spend their last days

Choosing a hospice in case he/she is not able to stay at home (hospice can also take place at home where medical staff would come, etc.)

What he/she wants to be said in their obituary

The choice of a funeral or memorial service

Wishes as to what music or songs, photos, or other things to have at the service

Preferences in asking for donations to be made and to whom instead of flowers

A list of who to notify of his/her death such as family, friends, and others such as banks, Social Security, creditors, etc.

Choices of the final disposition of their body such as cremation or burial

> If cremation is preferred, who should get ashes and where should they be spread

Wishes about donating their body or brain to science for research on dementia

Any other wishes your spouse may have that are not in his/her Will.

The plan needs to be witnessed by two witnesses and stored with the Will and other important or legal documents. If you have not considered donating his/her body or brain to science, the next topic will explain more about it.

54. BRAIN OR BODY DONATION TO SCIENCE

To some people, this may seem like a morbid idea; however, it is becoming more accepted and especially for those who would love to see a cure for dementia. Depending on your spouse's cognitive abilities, he/she can let you know if they would like to donate his/her brain after death so that scientific research can look for ways to cure dementia. Since your spouse would need to sign up for the donation program before he/she dies, you can request registration forms from your local chapter of donation service that you can locate by selecting your state on the Alzheimer's Association website.

There are also organizations or universities that your spouse can donate his/her whole body to science for research or be used for training medical professionals. The good thing about doing this is that when research or training is finished, they will perform a cremation at no cost to you. This is good to know if you do not wish to pay the high cost of a funeral. This is becoming a popular alternative to buying a burial plot and paying for a funeral. You can also plan on having a virtual memorial service on websites such as Never-Gone.com at NO cost.

Getting these things done should be part of your Care Plan, so you don't have to rush to get them done later. An attorney can help you with the correct forms for your state. If you cannot afford an attorney, there are advocates and social workers who can help as well as websites you can get free forms for each state. Doing all this can certainly be overwhelming and stressful for which the next topics will be of help to you and other caregivers taking care of your spouse.

STAGES OF DEMENTIA

54. EARLY STAGE

The early stages considered as mild because your spouse will still be able to function on their own with some mental or behavior issues. The early signs can be overlooked but family and close friends will start to notice that something is different. Since early symptoms were already listed, they will not be repeated. As discussed already, this is the time to get legal and financial matters in place.

In the earlier stages, he/she may not want your help as he/she may want to hang onto some independence. I suggest to always ask if he/she wants your help when he/she seems to be struggling with something.

55. MIDDLE STAGE

The middle stages considered to be moderate and can last for many years. As it progresses, your spouse will still be able to do daily activities but may need more help. It is important to understand what he/she can and can't do. Since the nerve cells in the brain become damaged, serious issues can arise such as:

- Losing long-term memories of personal history or information

- Mood swings that are more obvious
- Withdrawing from challenging situations
- Confusion that is more obvious about where things are, time, etc.
- Requiring help choosing clothing or making other decisions
- More consistent sleeping problems such being restless at night
- At risk of getting lost
- More significant behavior changes

56. LATE STAGE

Late-stage is also known as end-stage dementia and is classified as severe. Your spouse will require regular help and may not be able to do several tasks. As it worsens, personality changes may take place. Even though he/she may not be able to do as much during the late stage, there is still benefit from short visits with family, listening to relaxing music, or being gently touch. Here are some symptoms:

- Around-the-clock assistance may be needed
- Lack of memory of recent experiences or not knowing surroundings

- Having problems walking, sitting, and swallowing food
- Difficulty with talking or letting you know what he/she is feeling
- Can get infections easily with pneumonia as being common

With so much help needed, keeping resources and support for caregivers is absolutely necessary and here are some tips for you.

CAREGIVER TIPS

57. CAREGIVER HOTLINE

This is a number you need to put everywhere in your home. It is a 24-hour, 7-day a week including holidays hotline: HELPLINE 800.272.3900 or 711 for TRS

If it has not happened yet, there will come a time when you may need an answer that no one else can answer. That's when you can go to Alzheimer's Association's helpline. They have support for people living with the disease, caregivers, families, as well as the public. Here are some of their services:

- Master's-level care clinicians for confidential support in crisis assistance, discussion and education, decision-making assistance
- Find out about local programs and services
- Learn about the symptoms of Alzheimer's and other dementias
- General information on legal, financial, or care decisions, and treatment for managing symptoms
- Bilingual staff with translation service in more than 200 languages.

Now that you have someone to call for any questions, the following are some more important caregiver tips.

58. CAREGIVER MINDSET

Right from the start, try not to think of the worst-case scenario if your spouse has not been diagnosed. Until there is significant cause to believe your spouse has dementia, it is best not to discuss it that much with them as it can cause unnecessary worry and bring on more symptoms. This can be a real challenge for you and asking for help is something you must be able to do even if it is not something you are used to doing. Doing it all alone is not healthy for you and you must stay as healthy as possible to be able to care for someone you love. Even before you get a diagnosis, start asking other family members to help with whatever may be time-consuming such as grocery shopping. Another helpful thing before and after the diagnosis is journaling which is the next topic.

59. JOURNALING

Keeping a journal will be of great help in remembering things to do, tracking your spouse's symptoms, progression, concerns, and questions to ask the care team. I preferred using an electronic journal as it was much easier to search for things. If you do not have a computer, you can always write in a notebook and have someone on your team type it into an electronic journal on a daily or weekly basis.

Caregiving can become stressful but having a journal to keep information and to find patterns or triggers will help you in feeling more in control and less stressed. It will also help you be better equipped to solve problems and difficult behaviors. Having a dementia journal is an important caregiving tool. You can keep quick notes during the day in a notebook. A calendar notebook is best as it will have the day and times so you can jot a note next to the time that things happen. Using a computer or smartphone is fine too if it works best for you. You can get a free caregiver notebook template or a program for an electronic one at SpringWell.com (see Resources for a link). You will find it helpful in sharing information with family, other caregivers, or doctors. Here are some tips on what to track:

- A. Symptoms with type, severity, frequency, level of confusion

- B. Always note when a new symptom/behavior starts

- C. Challenging/difficult behaviors such as delusions, extreme anger, hallucinations, wandering

- D. Meals, drinks, and eating habits, what they ate and drank, appetite, snacks

- E. Toilet habits, accidents, need for incontinence products

- F. Safety issues: track what items your spouse may confuse with others to avoid accidents like brushing teeth with something other than toothpaste; it is similar to baby-proofing your home in that you would cover up things like the thermostat, outlets, etc. that they may try to use and break or get hurt.

- G. Things that will help your spouse find items such as marking drawers with the names or pictures of items in them

H. Medication list, effectiveness, and side effects

I. Information for doctor appointments such as falls, pain, fatigue, sleep problems, and incontinence

J. Write any questions for the doctor and take the notebook with to for telling the doctor about important issues, use the notebook to take notes.

Finding the time to keep the journal updated can be an issue. You may wish to contact a support group and the next topic will be of help for that.

60. CAREGIVER SUPPORT PROGRAMS

Caregiver Support Programs help caregivers reduce stress, make informed decisions, solve problems, and maintain overall emotional and physical health. SpringWell has a program that they charge for which is supposed to be 40 percent lower than others of its kind. You can call them at (617) 926-4100 x213 on Monday through Friday, 8:00 a.m. – 5:00 p.m., or email SolutionsInCare@springwell.com.

Alzheimer's Association has a support forum and other support features. They also have a Daily Care Plan for the person with dementia that you can set up for your spouse for doing activities, chores, etc. (see Resources for the link). Having your schedule is helpful and discussed next.

61. SCHEDULING

Having a schedule is critical. Your spouse may not be willing to go by your schedule so allow plenty of time for each aspect of his/her care. Try to make each part of the day for a certain activity such as bathing, meals, exercise, etc. Then try to keep to that time as much as possible. Be sure to schedule in when your caregiver alternate comes so you can have some time for yourself. Or schedule some time when your spouse is sleeping to catch up on your activities. It would be a good time to take classes online as in the next topic.

62. CAREGIVER CLASSES

Alzheimer's Association's website has free online programs that cover several topics, including AD basics and care strategies such as:

- 10 warning signs of AD
- Learn how AD affects the brain
- Managing caregiver stress
- Tips from the latest research

- Don't just hope for a cure, help us find one – volunteer for clinical trials
- You can sign up for news and events

63. CHOOSING MEDICAL AND SAFETY EQUIPMENT

Some websites have several ideas for the equipment that will help your spouse get around if his/her balance starts to be affected or walking becomes difficult. It is important to get your spouse outside when the weather is nice. It helps with depression and other symptoms. You want him/her to be safe and there is medical equipment to help and much of it is covered by insurance. Check with your insurance before buying and check with your doctor so they can order it and have the insurance billed.

One place to look is at the Alzheimer's Store (see Resources for a link). You can find an excellent variety of products for your spouse either by the stages of the early, middle, or late, by Category, by the most popular products, or by browsing it all. Some items are rather expensive and may not be covered by insurance so be sure to check before buying. Sometimes it may be worth the cost if you cannot find a certain item anywhere else. For example, I had no idea that you could buy stuffed pets that appear to be very real or little things for a person who needs something to do with their hands.

For a safety assessment checklist, go to Alzheimer's Association (see Resources for a link). It has questions for the caregiver and the patient. Depending on the answers there are considerations to review. Another issue is how this affects your emotions as discussed next.

64. IT IS NOT PERSONAL

At times it may seem like he/she does not love you anymore, but it is the disease that has changed him/her, and you cannot take it personally. Emotions may not be as evident in the later stages; however, every once in a while, your spouse may surprise you with a touching word or declaration of their love. They may show their love in subtle ways that you need to stop and appreciate. Usually, outbursts are a sign that something is not right, or they may be seeking your attention. Sometimes you get a gut feeling that something is not right as mentioned next.

65. SOMETHING IS NOT RIGHT

If you feel something is just not quite right, listen to your gut feeling. Your spouse may have had some early symptoms for some time and suddenly get worse. Since dementia can be a slow-growing condition, a sudden change could mean something else is going on. Other illnesses or problems can co-exist with dementia so sudden changes should be checked out. You are the expert in your spouse's behavior and health, so go with your intuition and seek medical help if something doesn't seem quite right. When your intuition and everything else seems disrupted, it is time for a break as discussed next.

66. TAKING BREAKS

You must get away from the house (and the spouse) if only for a few hours to have some time to contemplate matters, go to church, or visit with friends or family. I cannot emphasize enough that your health can decline slowly and before you know it, you will be in the hospital. There are many sad stories of the caregiver dying before the person with dementia because they overdid the self-sacrifice and did not take care of themselves. It can be a hard thing to do at times, but it can be done if you abide by what your body is telling you, be willing to ask for help often and follow your Care Plan which can be modified whenever it needs to be and if you need someone to step in for a time, I discuss this next.

67. SEEKING OTHER CARE

If for any reason you are not able to care for your spouse or those on your Care Team are telling you that you need to consider admitting your spouse into a facility, consider the alternatives. Some people will help you identify the need and help with the transition. If you just need him/her to stay somewhere temporarily, you can also investigate Respite Care which is a stay at a senior living community. Most have a variety of care levels, including assisted living, memory care, and skilled nursing. Remember that your love is not less just because you are not able to care for him/her anymore or need a break for a few weeks or months. You must think of your health as brought out in the next topic.

68. TAKING CARE OF YOURSELF

Please take it from one that knows...make time for you! To avoid caregiver burnout, it is an absolute necessity to take care of yourself first as the responsibility of caring for someone with dementia can be time-consuming and overwhelming at times. Being a caregiver can get to be harmful to you without being aware of it because you are so busy. Pick a time that your spouse is occupied or sleeping to do things that you like to do. I used to find that getting up early was the best time to focus on my interests. Some days things happen where you won't be able to take time for you, but if you can get just an hour or two every other day, it will help your frame of mind. Other ways of helping your frame of mind are covered next.

69. LEARNING THE LANGUAGE OF LOVE

During the five years that my husband had vascular dementia, I felt like I had to learn a new language. I called it the "Language of Love" because my love for him is what gave me the patience and the strength to deal with it. It was not easy at first because I did not have any support from family or friends. I had to remind myself of the love I had for him and how much he used to show his love to me. He had saved my life at one time when we first knew each other, and this was my way of showing how much I appreciated that. Unfortunately, love is not always enough. As part of the language of love, I am listing a few tips that should help you:

People can make the mistake of talking about your spouse as if he/she was not there right in front of him/her or talk to them like a child. Correct them if they do that and tell them to have respect as well as let him/her be part of conversations. Some of the

50 Things to Know

following tips can be put into your Care Plan so others will know how to approach your spouse.

- Before speaking to your spouse, find out when he/she is the most alert
- Make the room as quiet as possible by turning off TV or perhaps closing the door to keep out other noises
- Get his/her full attention without being hungry or tired
- Get close enough so they can hear well and be at the same level
- Use body language that does not depict being in a hurry and make eye contact
- Keep questions short and simple on one subject
- Speak slow, calm without being too loud but clear
- Use humor to make light of misunderstandings
- Try to phrase questions to have a brief answer or just a yes or no answer
- If they do not understand, rephrase the question, or break it up into parts
- Allow plenty of time for them to answer

- Pay attention to body language as they may not have words but can show you
- If having a good day and he/she can express worries or problems, show you are listening
- Touching his/her hand or shoulder or giving a light hug is usually very much welcomed.
- Try to keep any negative attitude or comments when frustrated to yourself as it can cause your spouse to become upset.

70. ANGER MANAGEMENT

Your spouse may become angry from getting confused, over-stimulated, being overwhelmed, lonely, or bored can cause anger or aggression.

Here are some tips that may help if they are not displaying severe anger that may be dangerous:

- Put on some soft soothing music they like
- Give a stuffed pet or doll they like
- Sooth with gentle touching
- Speak in a calm voice with reassurances
- Distract with an activity or routine they like to do

Determine how angry he/she may be to see if it is best to leave them alone to calm down or not. If anger symptoms are getting out of control or often, speak to the doctor about getting certain medications that can help.

71. HANDLING MISBELIEFS OR DELUSIONS

Part of the language of love is not correcting your spouse's misbeliefs or delusions because it is not worth the argument that may ensue. It will take a little practice to recognize when he/she may be seeing things that are not there or believing something that is not true. When my husband had a delusion that we were in an airplane instead of a hospital, I would go along with him. When I was on the way to talk to the doctor, I told him I had to go see the pilot. When I got back, I told him we were about to land, and the flight attendant was coming to take him out of the plane and take him to a different plane.

I knew he felt more comfortable in an airplane than anywhere, so I made that up when he was going to be transferred to a nursing home. It was shortly after he had surgery to amputate his leg and dementia increased tremendously for a time as it can do after having anesthesia. When he was transferred to a nursing home to recover, he would not stay in bed and kept the nurses running when he would try to get up and set off the alarm. The doctor prescribed a medication called Aricept (Donepezil) which was a blessing. It calmed him down and turned him into the sweetest old man. Another thing that calmed him down was being around family.

72. BE AROUND FAMILY

Family can be so important to your spouse, especially in the early and middle stage. In the late stage, he/she may not seem to notice they are there or know who they are, but I feel it is still important for them to have loved ones around.

Eventually, my husband and I moved in with my son and his family which was helpful. He perked up at being around his grandchildren and our son. Then our daughter came and stayed for a few months and he loved having two of me as he would get us mixed up. My other son came to visit as well as other family and I could tell he thrived on their attention.

There is a cute story about when our grandson met his Grandpa for the first time about three months before he died. The little guy was so intrigued by his Grandpa as he was explaining to him that he was going to love airplanes someday because he had aviation fuel in his blood. Our grandson's eyes got enormous and at only 11 days old, he smiled as if he knew what Grandpa was saying. He is now 14 years

50 Things to Know

old and wants to learn to fly as he loves airplanes and so does his 17-year-old sister.

This was part of my 'silver lining' of seeing the good things of his condition as discussed next.

73. THE SILVER LINING CONCLUSION

When I say that I began to see the silver lining in the way my husband had become, it was mostly because my attitude improved when I was able to have more help. I know it helped him to cope with dementia and other health problems better. As explained before, his deminer changed when we were around family more.

Two days before he died, it was a beautiful spring day in May, so I rolled him in his wheelchair out to the patio of the hospice. I heard airplanes flying overhead and looked up to watch them. There was a small airport close by and as I looked up, I heard him say "Cessna 150." He was not looking up at the sky. He had a clear moment and identified what type of airplane it was as it flew overhead. I looked up and sure enough, it was a Cessna 150. He identified it by the sound of its engine as he had done for years before. I will hold that memory as well as many others dear to my heart.

I feel that my husband was fortunate to have died before getting significantly worse. He could have suffered for more years and I was thankful that my prayers were answered. He most likely had another stroke. My heart goes out to anyone who is dealing with taking care of a spouse with possible long-term Alzheimer's.

May you be blessed with some quality time with your spouse and God bless you for taking such loving care of him/her.

OTHER RESOURCES:

Websites on Dementia:

Aging Care has a forum to ask questions and free senior care guides: https://www.agingcare.com
Alzheimer's Association: https://www.alz.org/
Alzheimer's Association National Early-Stage Advisory Group (ESAG): https://www.alz.org/about/leadership/early-stage-advisory-group
Alzheimer's Association Care Planning: Dementia Care Planning | Alzheimer's Association
Alzheimer's Association Our Personal Facts and Insights form: https://www.alz.org/media/Documents/personal-facts-insights.pdf
Alzheimer's Association Safety Assessment Checklist: www.alz.org/media/Documents/safety-assess-checklist.pdf
Alzheimer's Association Daily Care Plan: https://www.alz.org/help-support/caregiving/daily-care/daily-care-plan
Alzheimer's Navigator (part of the Alzheimer's Association): https://www.alzheimersnavigator.org/

Alzheimer's Net: https://www.alzheimers.net/

Alzheimer's Organization: https://www.alzheimersorganization.org/

Alzheimer's Organization (UK) "This is Me" form: www.alzheimers.org.uk/sites/default/files/migrate/downloads/this_is_me.pdf

Daily Caring: https://dailycaring.com/keeping-a-dementia-journal-makes-caregiving-easier-7-things-to-track/

Caregiver Contract Agreement: https://www.formstemplates.com/contract or https://www.lawdepot.com/contracts (you can get a free trial but need to cancel unless you want to pay a monthly fee)

Mayo Clinic: https://www.mayoclinic.org/diseases-conditions/dementia/

More Than Cognition: https://morethancognition.neurologyreviews.com/

National Caregiver's Library – Document organizer and many other forms and documents: www.caregiverslibrary.org/Portals/0/ChecklistsandForms_CaregiverDocumentOrganizer.pdf

Very Well Health: https://www.verywellhealth.com/types-of-dementia-98770?print

The Alzheimer's Store:
https://www.alzstore.com/shop-alzheimers-stores/2054.htm

SpringWell Caregiver Notebook:
https://springwell.com/resource/caregiver-notebook/

SpringWell Caregiver Support:
http://springwell2.wpengine.com/service/caregiver-support/

Videos About Dementia:

Experience 12 Minutes in Alzheimer's Dementia:
https://www.youtube.com/watch?v=LL_Gq7Shc-Y

Alzheimer's Association – Voices of Alzheimer's:
https://youtu.be/0mzCJ80sDRs

READ OTHER 50 THINGS TO KNOW BOOKS

50 Things to Know to Get Things Done Fast: Easy Tips for Success

50 Things to Know About Going Green: Simple Changes to Start Today

50 Things to Know to Live a Happy Life Series

50 Things to Know to Organize Your Life: A Quick Start Guide to Declutter, Organize, and Live Simply

50 Things to Know About Being a Minimalist: Downsize, Organize, and Live Your Life

50 Things to Know About Speed Cleaning: How to Tidy Your Home in Minutes

50 Things to Know About Choosing the Right Path in Life

50 Things to Know to Get Rid of Clutter in Your Life: Evaluate, Purge, and Enjoy Living

50 Things to Know About Journal Writing: Exploring Your Innermost Thoughts & Feelings

50 Things to Know

50 Things to Know

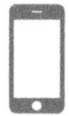

Stay up to date with new releases on Amazon:

https://amzn.to/2VPNGr7

50 Things to Know

We'd love to hear what you think about our content! Please leave your honest review of this book on Amazon and Goodreads. We appreciate your positive and constructive feedback. Thank you.

www.ingramcontent.com/pod-product-compliance
Lightning Source LLC
Chambersburg PA
CBHW070425220526
45466CB00004B/1550